Peripheral Neuropathy Diet & Cookbook

Your Comprehensive Guide to Managing Neuropathy Symptoms With Dietary and Lifestyle Strategies.

Title:
Peripheral Neuropathy Diet & Cookbook

Subtitle

Your Comprehensive Guide to Managing Neuropathy Symptoms With Dietary and Lifestyle Strategies.

Copyright © 2023 by (Reynold Morissette Ph.D.)

Printed in the United States of America.

ISBN: 9798864805152

TABLE OF CONTENT

INTRODUCTION

Millions of people worldwide suffer from peripheral neuropathy, which is defined as damage to the peripheral nerves that carry messages from the central nervous system to the rest of the body. These nerves, which regulate our sensations and motor abilities, are crucial to day-to-day functioning. When they are harmed, a variety of symptoms can appear, ranging from tingling and numbness to severe pain and muscle weakness, making even the most straightforward actions difficult.

Living with peripheral neuropathy can be difficult and frequently uncomfortable. It can result from several factors, including diabetes, autoimmune illnesses, vitamin deficiencies, drugs, and more, and it affects people of all ages and socioeconomic backgrounds. Despite the importance of pharmacological interventions and therapies in controlling this condition, diet plays a key role in symptom relief and promoting nerve function.

Your guide to comprehending the critical link between what you eat and how it affects your peripheral nerves is this book, "Peripheral Neuropathy Diet." This book, which was written by a qualified nutritionist, is intended to give you the information and resources you need to take charge of your health. It is a comprehensive tool to assist you in making informed food decisions and lifestyle changes that can supplement your ongoing medical treatment and enhance your quality of life rather than a one-size-fits-all approach.

You will learn more about the complex connection between nutrition and peripheral neuropathy in the pages that follow. You will learn which nutrients are crucial for nerve health, which meals can encourage recovery, and which foods to stay away from if your symptoms get worse. We will examine how blood sugar management affects neuropathy management, especially for people with diabetes.

You will come across helpful recommendations, meal plans, recipes, and guidance along the way to assist you in choosing the best diet for you. We'll talk about the possible advantages of supplements and how to properly include them in your routine. Additionally, this book won't just concentrate on diet; it will also cover larger lifestyle modifications like exercise, stress reduction, and the value of getting enough sleep that can help you manage your neuropathy.

It is important to keep in mind that each person's experience with peripheral neuropathy is different, even though this book offers helpful insights into how to manage the condition through diet and lifestyle adjustments. Before making any big dietary or lifestyle changes, always check with your doctor. You can use this book as a supplement to their advice.

Let's start this adventure together and discover how the Peripheral Neuropathy Diet can help you regain control and improve your general well-being. By the time you finish reading this book, you will have the information and techniques necessary to develop a unique plan for controlling your peripheral neuropathy, one mouthful at a time.

CHAPTER 1: UNDERSTANDING PERIPHERAL NEUROPATHY

What Is Peripheral Neuropathy?

Damage to the peripheral nerves, which are in charge of transferring impulses between the brain, spinal cord, and the rest of the body, results in peripheral neuropathy, a complicated and frequently painful medical condition. These nerves serve as our body's "highways of communication," enabling us to receive sensations, command our motions, and manage our bodily processes. This crucial network is disturbed when peripheral neuropathy arises.

The term "peripheral" refers to the nerves that are not a part of the brain and spinal cord, which make up the central nervous system. A broad word for nerve injury or malfunction is neuropathy. As a result, peripheral neuropathy refers to the nerve damage that affects the arms, hands, legs, and feet. This can result in a wide range of distressing symptoms that vary in form and degree and have a varied impact on every person.

Causes and Risk Factors

Effective management and prevention of peripheral neuropathy depend on an understanding of its origins and risk factors. There are several underlying causes for this syndrome, including:

1. **Diabetes:** One of the most frequent causes is diabetic neuropathy, which results from long-term nerve damage brought on by high blood sugar levels.

2. **Autoimmune Diseases:** Rheumatoid arthritis, lupus, and Guillain-Barré

syndrome are autoimmune diseases that can cause neuropathy.

3. Illnesses: HIV, hepatitis, and Lyme disease are a few viral and bacterial infections that can harm your nerves.

4. Medication: Neuropathy is a potential adverse effect of some drugs, particularly those used in chemotherapy.

5. Chemicals, heavy metals, and environmental pollutants can harm neurons when they are exposed.

6. Alcoholism: Drinking too much alcohol
   can damage your nerves and cause
   alcoholic neuropathy.

7. Nutritional Deficiencies: Neuropathy
   can be brought on by a deficiency in
   important nutrients including the B
   vitamins, particularly B1 (thiamine),
   B6 (pyridoxine), B9 (folate), and B12
   (cobalamin).

8. Genetics: Some people may be
   predisposed to neuropathy due to
   certain genetic conditions.

9. Trauma and Injury: Direct nerve injury can result from physical trauma or accidents.

10. Aging: People are increasingly prone to neuropathy as they get older.

For effective management and tailored treatment, determining the underlying cause is essential. Peripheral neuropathy risk can also be increased by risk factors such as family history, current medical problems, and lifestyle choices.

Symptoms and Diagnosis

Numerous symptoms, varying in intensity and appearance, might be a sign of peripheral neuropathy. Typical signs include:

- Feeling of pins and needles in the affected area due to numbness or tingling.
- A burning or shooting pain is frequently described as being extremely painful.
- Having weak muscles makes it difficult to balance or use fine motor abilities.
- Coordination loss: Difficulty walking or executing other coordinated-demanding tasks.
- Skin that is sensitive to touch or temperature changes may react

abnormally to changes in temperature.

- Nail alterations, hair loss, and dry, brittle, or thinning skin are all examples of changes to the skin, hair, and nails.

Numerous diagnostic tests, a thorough medical history, and a physical examination are frequently used to identify peripheral neuropathy. Among these examinations are electromyography (EMG), blood tests to measure nutrition and glucose levels, nerve conduction studies, and occasionally imaging examinations to rule out structural problems.

The Role of Diet and Nutrition

The impact of diet and nutrition on peripheral neuropathy is a central theme of this book. Proper nutrition plays a significant role in preventing and managing neuropathy, particularly when it is related to diabetes, alcohol abuse, or nutritional deficiencies. Nutrients like B vitamins, antioxidants, and essential fatty acids are crucial for nerve health. Additionally, blood sugar control through diet can help mitigate symptoms and prevent further nerve damage in those with diabetic neuropathy.

This book will explore how specific nutrients and dietary choices can influence the progression of peripheral neuropathy, offering guidance on crafting a neuropathy-friendly diet that supports nerve health and overall well-being. By understanding the underlying mechanisms and exploring the dietary strategies provided in this book, you will be better equipped to take control of your health and improve your quality of life while managing peripheral neuropathy. This book's main focus is the effect of diet and nutrition on peripheral neuropathy. Especially when it is linked to diabetes, alcoholism, or nutritional deficits, proper diet is crucial for both avoiding and controlling neuropathy. The health of the nerves depends on nutrients including B vitamins, antioxidants, and vital fatty acids. Additionally, diet-based blood sugar management can lessen symptoms and stop additional nerve damage in people with diabetic neuropathy.

This book will examine how particular nutrients and dietary decisions might affect the development of peripheral neuropathy and will provide advice on how to create a diet that is supportive of nerve health and general well-being while also being neuropathy-friendly.

You will be better able to take charge of your health and enhance your quality of life while managing peripheral neuropathy if you comprehend the underlying causes and investigate the dietary recommendations included in this book.

CHAPTER 2: THE BASICS OF NUTRITION AND NEUROPATHY

A complicated illness known as peripheral neuropathy affects the peripheral nerves' capacity to send messages from the central nervous system to the body's extremities. While medicinal interventions are essential for controlling neuropathy, nutrition also becomes a key component of the all-encompassing care strategy. The groundwork for comprehending the fundamental concepts of nutrition and how they relate to neuropathy will be laid forth in this chapter.

The Importance of a Well-Balanced Diet

A complex disorder called peripheral neuropathy affects how well the peripheral nerves can communicate with the body's extremities and the central nervous system. Nutrition also appears as a key component in the entire care plan, even though medical therapies are essential for controlling neuropathy. This chapter will establish the groundwork for comprehending nutrition's basic principles and how they relate to neuropathy.

- Proteins: The building block of nerve regeneration, proteins are crucial for muscle function and tissue repair.

- Carbs: Carbohydrates provide the body energy, and the correct kinds of carbohydrates can help control blood sugar levels, a crucial aspect of managing neuropathy.

- Fats: Good fats are essential for keeping cell membranes, which are necessary for nerve activity, in good condition.

- Fiber: Fiber helps with digestion and may help with blood sugar regulation.

- Numerous vitamins and minerals have specific functions in maintaining the health of the nervous system.

- Antioxidants: These substances defend cells against oxidative injury and inflammation, which can result in nerve damage.

Knowing the value of eating a healthy, balanced diet will enable you to plan your meals and snacks wisely, thus promoting the health of your peripheral nerves.

Key Nutrients for Nerve Health

It's crucial to concentrate on particular nutrients that have a direct impact on nerve health when treating peripheral neuropathy. These essential nutrients are broken down into numerous groups:

Vitamins

- B vitamins, such as thiamine (vitamin B1), pyridoxine (vitamin B6), folate (vitamin B9), and cobalamin (vitamin B12), are necessary for healthy nerve function and can lessen or avoid neuropathic symptoms.

Minerals

- Magnesium: Magnesium is necessary for the movement of nerves and muscles.

- Calcium: Calcium is essential for the movement of nerve impulses and the contraction of muscles.

- Zinc: This mineral promotes healthy neurological and immunological systems.

- Copper: Copper is essential for the development of myelin, the covering that protects nerve fibers.

Antioxidants

- Vitamin C is a potent antioxidant that can aid in lowering oxidative stress, which can lead to nerve damage.

- Vitamin E: Another antioxidant that guards against harm to the membranes of nerve cells.

- Selenium: Selenium helps the body's defenses against free radicals.

Essential Fatty Acids

- Omega-3 Fatty Acids: These beneficial fats can lower inflammation and support the structure and operation of nerve cells.

Amino Acids

- L-carnitine: By helping nerve cells produce energy, this amino acid may reduce the symptoms of neuropathic pain.

- L-glutamine: It contributes to the operation of neurotransmitters and can support the health of the nerves.

The first step in designing your diet to properly treat peripheral neuropathy is to understand these important nutrients and their roles in maintaining the health of your nerves.

The Impact of Blood Sugar Control

Controlling blood sugar is essential for treating peripheral neuropathy, especially in cases when diabetes is involved. High blood sugar levels can wreak havoc on the nervous system and make neuropathic symptoms worse. Therefore, it is crucial to control neuropathy while keeping blood sugar levels steady.

Important considerations for controlling blood sugar include:

- Dietary Glycemic Index: By being aware of a food's glycemic index, you can pick carbs that won't significantly raise your blood sugar levels.

- Balanced Meals: Consuming an appropriate amount of carbohydrates, proteins, and fats will assist in maintaining blood sugar levels at each meal.

- Regular Monitoring: As directed by a healthcare professional, routine blood sugar monitoring is crucial for managing diabetes.

Dietary Glycemic Index: By being aware of a food's glycemic index, you can pick carbs that won't significantly raise your blood sugar levels.

Balanced Meals: Consuming an appropriate amount of carbohydrates, proteins, and fats will assist in maintaining blood sugar levels at each meal.

Regular Monitoring: As directed by a healthcare professional, routine blood sugar monitoring is crucial for managing diabetes.

CHAPTER 3: CRAFTING YOUR NEUROPATHY-FRIENDLY DIET

Peripheral neuropathy, a condition that disrupts the normal functioning of the peripheral nervous system, can be challenging to manage. The symptoms, ranging from tingling and numbness to sharp pain and muscle weakness, can significantly impact your daily life. While medical treatments and therapies are important aspects of managing neuropathy, your diet plays a pivotal role in symptom control and overall well-being. In this chapter, we will explore how to create a neuropathy-focused diet, encompassing dietary guidelines, sample meal plans, and the importance of portion control.

Creating a Neuropathy-Focused Meal Plan

Your nutritional strategy for treating this ailment is built on a meal plan specifically designed for people with neuropathy. It requires careful food selection, meal planning, and portion control to ensure that you provide your body with the nutrients it needs while reducing the possibility of symptom flare.

Dietary Guidelines

Dietary recommendations serve as a guide for creating a menu that promotes nerve health and lessens the effects of peripheral neuropathy. These recommendations offer guidance on choosing the proper nutrients and keeping a balanced diet that is supportive of symptom alleviation and general well-being.

Balanced Macronutrients: It's important to strike a balance between your intake of carbohydrates, proteins, and fats. This equilibrium helps to maintain steady blood sugar levels and provides the essential nutrients for healthy neuronal function.

Prioritizing foods that are high in nutrients is crucial.

These foods are full of antioxidants, vitamins, and minerals that are essential for nerve healing and maintenance. Your diet should be built around them.

Regular Meals: Consuming food at regular intervals helps control blood sugar levels and prevents dramatic swings that could exacerbate neuropathy symptoms.

Sample Meal Plans

Examples of meal plans offer helpful advice on how to organize your everyday eating habits. These menus serve as examples of how to apply dietary recommendations to your daily life and as a springboard for creating your customized meal plan. They include alternatives for breakfast, lunch, dinner, and snacks, all of which were created with the management of neuropathy in mind.

Day 1:

Breakfast

- Whole-grain toast

- Fresh orange slices

- Scrambled eggs with spinach and tomatoes

- Herbal tea

Lunch

- Quinoa.

- Salad of grilled chicken breast with cherry tomatoes, mixed greens, and balsamic vinaigrette.

- A small serving of low-fat yogurt.

Dinner

- Steamed broccoli

- Brown rice

- Baked salmon with lemon and dill

- Mixed berries with a drizzle of honey
  for dessert

Snack

Baby carrots with hummus

Day 2:

Breakfast

- Sliced banana.

- Green tea.

- Greek yogurt with honey and walnuts.

Lunch

- Whole-grain roll.

- A small serving of fruit salad.

- Lentil and vegetable soup.

Dinner

- Brown rice.

- Tofu and a variety of veggies are stir-fried in a low-sodium sauce.

- For dessert, serve sliced strawberries with a garnish of dark chocolate shavings.

Snack

- A handful of mixed nuts.

Day 3:

Breakfast

- Herbal tea.

- Fresh berries with nut butter drizzled over oatmeal.

Lunch

- salad of spinach dressed in balsamic vinaigrette.

- cottage cheese with less fat.

- Sandwich made with turkey and avocado on whole-grain bread.

Dinner

- Quinoa.

- For dessert, a small portion of peach slices.

- Grilled shrimp with garlic and herbs.

- Steamed asparagus.

Snack

- Cucumber slices with tzatziki sauce.

Day 4:

Breakfast

- Waffles made of whole grains served with kiwi slices and Greek yogurt.

- Green tea.

Lunch

- Whole-grain pita bread.

- A small serving of mixed fruit.

- Chickpea and vegetable stew.

Dinner

- Mixed berries with a dollop of whipped cream for dessert.

- Baked chicken breast with rosemary.

- Roasted sweet potatoes.

- Sautéed kale.

Snack

- Sea salt sprinkled on top of edamame.

Day 5:

Breakfast

- Whole-grain toast.

- Sliced strawberries.

- Herbal tea.

- Spinach and mushroom omelet.

Lunch

- feta cheese and roasted veggie quinoa salad.

- a little yogurt with reduced fat.

Dinner

- Baked cod with lemon and herbs.
- Dessert is sliced mango with honey drizzling.
- Steamed broccoli.
- Brown rice.

Snack

Hummus and sliced bell peppers.

Day 6:

Breakfast

- Greek yogurt with chopped almonds, honey, and banana slices.
- Green tea.

Lunch

- Whole-grain roll.
- A small serving of fruit salad.
- Lentil and vegetable soup.

Dinner

- Brown rice.
- Tofu and a variety of veggies are stir-fried in a low-sodium sauce.

- For dessert, serve sliced strawberries with a garnish of dark chocolate shavings.

Snack

- a bunch of different nuts.

Day 7:

Breakfast

- Fresh berries with nut butter drizzled over oatmeal.
- Herbal tea.

Lunch

- Low-fat cottage cheese.

- Sandwich made with turkey and avocado on whole-grain bread.
- salad of spinach dressed in balsamic vinaigrette.

Dinner

- Steamed asparagus.
- Quinoa.
- Grilled shrimp with garlic and herbs.
- A small serving of sliced peaches for dessert.

Snack

- Sliced cucumbers with tzatziki sauce.

Day 8:
Breakfast

- Sliced papaya

- Green tea

- Scrambled eggs with diced bell peppers and onions

- Whole-grain toast

Lunch

- Cucumber, cherry tomatoes, and feta cheese in a quinoa salad.

- A little Greek yogurt serve.

Dinner

- Steamed broccoli.

- Wild rice.

- Grilled salmon with a lemon-herb marinade.

- Mixed berries with a drizzle of honey for dessert.

Snack

Sliced apple with almond butter

Day 9:

Breakfast

- Herbal tea

- Chia seeds, fresh berries, and a drizzle of honey added to overnight oats.

Lunch

- Whole-grain roll

- Low-fat cottage cheese

- Grilled chicken breast, cherry tomatoes, and a vinaigrette dressing on top of a salad of spinach and mixed greens.

Dinner

- Roasted sweet potatoes.

- Sautéed kale.

- Baked tilapia with a garlic and herb crust.

- Sliced mango with a dollop of whipped cream for dessert.

Snack

- Sliced cucumbers with hummus

Day 10:

Breakfast

- Pancakes made with whole grains, fresh blueberries, and yogurt on top.

- Green tea

Lunch

- Brown rice

- Lentil and vegetable stir-fry with tofu.

- A small serving of fruit salad.

Dinner

- Steamed asparagus

- Quinoa

- Grilled turkey burgers with avocado and mixed greens

- A small serving of mixed fruit for

  dessert

Snack

- A handful of mixed nuts

These sample meal plans offer variety and flavor while adhering to dietary guidelines for neuropathy management. Feel free to modify them according to your preferences and dietary needs, ensuring that they align with your specific requirements.

Portion Control

Controlling your portions is essential for controlling neuropathy, especially if you have diabetes. Without bringing on sharp surges in blood sugar, it helps maintain consistent nutrient intake. It is impossible to stress the importance of portion control in your effort to effectively treat the symptoms of neuropathy.

The following are some portion-controlling techniques:

1. Use Smaller Plates: To automatically minimize portion sizes, choose smaller plates and bowls. You may be able to eat

fewer portions and still feel satisfied if you perceive your plate as being full.

2. Measure Servings: To precisely measure your portions, buy measuring glasses and a food scale. This is crucial for foods like grains, pasta, and proteins in particular.

3. Be Conscious of Snacking: To avoid overeating, keep portioned snack options close at hand. Small containers of nuts and fruits or prepackaged snacks might help limit quantities.

4. Consume Food Slowly: By taking your time and savoring each bite, you can

learn to detect fullness and avoid overeating.

5. Divide restaurant servings with a dining companion or immediately package half of the meal to take home when eating out.

6. Don't Take Second Helpings: Don't take second helpings because they can result in consuming too many calories.

7. Engage in Mindful Eating: Pay attention to your food. To enjoy your meal more and avoid overeating, pay close attention to the flavors and textures of your food.

8. Keep Food Journals: Record your meals and portion sizes in a food journal. You can do this to maintain accountability and spot any tendencies of excessive consumption.

Food Choices and Substitutions

Choosing the right foods and substituting them when necessary is a crucial part of the dietary management of peripheral neuropathy. This section will look at different food groups and ingredients that may be especially helpful for people with neuropathy. These options can lessen pain caused by peripheral neuropathy, control blood sugar levels, and enhance nerve health.

Fiber-Rich Foods

A neuropathy-friendly diet must include foods high in fiber. They have several benefits:

- Blood Sugar Stabilization: Foods containing soluble fiber, such as oats, lentils, and some fruits, can help manage blood sugar levels. This is essential for patients who suffer neuropathy, especially if diabetes is the underlying reason.

- Digestive Health: Fiber promotes healthy digestion and helps ease symptoms like constipation, which can exacerbate neuropathic pain.

- Weight management: Retaining a healthy weight helps ease nerve pressure and lessen the chance of neuropathy problems. By encouraging a sensation of fullness and discouraging overeating, fiber-rich foods can aid in weight management.

Fiber-rich food options:

- Brown rice, quinoa, and whole wheat are examples of whole grains.

- vegetables including kale, spinach, and broccoli.

- legumes such as chickpeas, black beans, and lentils.

- fruits such as berries, pears, and apples.

- almonds, chia seeds, and flaxseeds, among other nuts and seeds.

Lean Proteins

For the health of the nervous system and general well-being, protein is a crucial nutrient. Lean protein sources are healthier options for people with neuropathy since they include fewer harmful fats. Lean protein advantages include:

- Proteins give the body essential amino acids, which serve as the building blocks of neural tissue. A sufficient protein intake can help in nerve regeneration and repair.

- Blood Sugar Control: Meals high in protein can help maintain blood sugar levels, lowering the chance of surges in neuropathic pain.

- Maintaining muscular mass and strength is crucial for people with neuropathy because it improves balance and lowers the chance of falling.

Lean protein sources:

- Skinless chicken (chicken, turkey).

- lean pork and beef slices.

- Fish (especially fatty fish like salmon and trout for omega-3 fatty acids).

- Tempeh and tofu (for plant-based options).

- Legumes (beans, lentils, and chickpeas).

Complex Carbohydrates

It is essential to choose complex carbs over simple ones for treating peripheral neuropathy. Complex carbs provide long-lasting energy without spiking blood sugar levels because they break down slowly. The benefits of complex carbs are as follows:

Consistent Energy: These carbs help to maintain steady energy levels throughout the day by gradually releasing glucose into the bloodstream.

Blood sugar control: By reducing the highs and lows that can cause neuropathic discomfort, a varied carbohydrate-based diet can regulate blood sugar.

Numerous complex carbs are high in fiber, which aids in digestion and promotes blood sugar stability.

Complex carbohydrate sources:

- Oats, whole wheat pasta, and other whole grains.

- Sweet potatoes and carrots are examples of root veggies.

- Legumes such as black beans and lentils.

- Vegetables like broccoli and squash.

Healthy Fats

The health of your nerves and general well-being depend on healthy fats. Particularly renowned for their anti-inflammatory qualities, omega-3 fatty acids can be helpful for neuropathy. Healthy fats have several benefits, such as:

- Omega-3 fatty acids, which are present in fatty fish and flaxseeds, have anti-inflammatory effects that may aid in relieving neuropathic pain.

- Healthy fats are crucial parts of the membranes that surround nerve cells, ensuring their well-being and proper operation.

- Cardiovascular Health: As people with neuropathy are more likely to experience heart-related problems, healthy fats must support heart health.

Healthy fat sources:

- Nuts and seeds.
- Avocado.
- Olive oil.

- Fatty fish, such as sardines, mackerel, and salmon.

- Both chia and flax seeds.

Sugar Reduction

One of the most important components of controlling neuropathy is reducing sugar intake. High sugar intake might cause blood sugar to rise and aggravate symptoms related to the nerves. Take into account the following tactics to cut back on sugar:

- Limiting Added Sugars: Limit your intake of sweetened beverages, processed foods, and sugar-sweetened desserts.

- Natural Sweeteners: As an alternative to refined sugar, try using natural sweeteners like stevia or monk fruit.

- Balanced Carbohydrates: To reduce the rate at which sugar enters the system, combine carbohydrates with protein and good fats.

- Portion Control: Be mindful of portion sizes when consuming foods with natural sugars, like fruits.

Special Considerations for Dietary Restrictions

It's crucial to realize that persons with peripheral neuropathy may have special dietary restrictions or preferences. These can include food allergies, sensitivities, or dietary choices (e.g., vegetarian or vegan) (e.g., vegetarian or vegan). It's vital to alter the neuropathy-friendly diet to accommodate these constraints. Seek suitable substitutions, and check with a healthcare physician or a qualified dietitian if you have particular dietary needs.

CHAPTER 4: FOODS TO EMBRACE AND AVOID

Foods that support peripheral neuropathy are essential for treating this ailment successfully. You may improve your general well-being, have a good impact on the health of your nerves, and relieve symptoms by making deliberate and well-informed food decisions. We will look at several foods in this chapter that you should embrace and include in your diet regularly. We'll go over the benefits of these foods for managing neuropathy as well as some advice on how to enjoy them.

Neuropathy-Friendly Foods

Peripheral neuropathy-friendly foods are those that are rich in essential nutrients, vitamins, and minerals that can support nerve health and minimize inflammation. Here are some key categories of such foods:

Nuts and Seeds

Nuts and seeds are nutrient powerhouses that provide several advantages for people with peripheral neuropathy:

- Contains vitamin E, a powerful antioxidant that shields nerves from oxidative stress.

- contain B vitamins, such as B6 and B12, which are essential for the health of the nervous system.

- Offer wholesome fats like omega-3 fatty acids, which can lower inflammation and enhance the health of your nerves.

- Low in carbs and beneficial for blood sugar stabilization.

Recommended options: Flaxseeds, chia seeds, Almonds, walnuts, and sunflower seeds.

Leafy Greens

Leafy greens are nutrient-dense and have many benefits for nerve health, including:

- Especially B vitamins like folate and B6, which are crucial for nerve function, are abundant in vitamins.
- rich in antioxidants that fight oxidative damage, including vitamins C and K.
- fiber-rich, which helps to maintain steady blood sugar levels.
- They are low in calories and a great option for weight maintenance.

Recommended options: Swiss chard, Spinach, kale, and collard greens.

Lean Meats and Fish

Exceptional sources of high-quality protein and vital elements that support nerve health include lean meats and fish:

- Rich in vitamin B12, which is essential for nerve repair and function.

- To maintain healthy muscles and general well-being, give protein.

- Include vital amino acids that serve as the foundation for nerve tissue.

- Omega-3 fatty acids are abundant, and they have anti-inflammatory characteristics.

Recommended options: Skinless chicken, lean beef cuts, salmon, mackerel, and trout.

Whole Grains

Whole grains provide several nutritional benefits and can aid with blood sugar stabilization:

- Rich in dietary fiber, which slows the absorption of sugars and reduces blood sugar spikes.

- Contains essential B vitamins, particularly thiamine, which supports nerve function.

- Provide sustained energy, promoting overall vitality.

- Support digestive health, which is essential for nutrient absorption.

Recommended options: Quinoa, brown rice, whole wheat pasta, and oats.

Low-Glycemic Fruits

Low-glycemic fruits are those with little effect on blood sugar levels:

- Essential vitamins and antioxidants that protect nerve cells are present.

- Fiber content is high, which delays sugar absorption.

- Aid in the regulation of blood sugar levels, lowering the risk of neuropathy-related problems.

Recommended options: Berries (such as blueberries and strawberries), apples, pears, and cherries are all examples of fruits.

Foods to Limit or Avoid

Certain dietary choices can aggravate peripheral neuropathy. It is critical to be conscious of the meals you consume to effectively manage and lessen its symptoms. Here are some dietary groups to limit or avoid:

Processed Foods

Processed meals are often heavy in artificial additives, preservatives, and unhealthy fats, making them harmful to people suffering from peripheral neuropathy. These meals frequently lack vital nutrients, which can contribute to inflammation and poor blood sugar regulation. It is critical to reduce or eliminate:

- Canned soups and sauces

- Fast food

- Sugary cereals

- Frozen dinners

- Processed meats (sausages, hot dogs).

- Sugary and artificially flavored beverages.

Sugary Snacks

Excess sugar consumption can cause blood sugar spikes and inflammation, both of which can exacerbate peripheral neuropathy symptoms. Sugary treats, such as: should be limited or avoided.

- Sweetened cereals.

- Pastries and baked goods.

- Soda and other sugary beverages.

- Candy and chocolate bars.

- Sugary snacks like chips and cookies.

Excess Sodium

A high-sodium diet can cause elevated blood pressure and fluid retention, which can exacerbate neuropathy symptoms, especially in people who have underlying diseases such as hypertension. Excess sodium foods to avoid include:

- Fast food items high in salt

- Canned soups and vegetables

- Instant noodles

- Processed meats (ham, bacon)

- High-sodium condiments (soy sauce, teriyaki sauce)

Trans Fats

Trans fats are synthetic fats present in a variety of processed and fried meals. They can cause inflammation and impair cardiovascular health, both of which can have a detrimental impact on neuropathy. Avoid or limit your consumption of trans-fat-containing foods, such as:

- Margarine and butter replacements are available.

- Commercially prepared baked goods (donuts, cookies, pastries).

- Fast food that is fried (French fries, fried chicken).

- Some packaged treats (microwave popcorn).

- Desserts packaged in hydrogenated oils.

CHAPTER 5: SUPPLEMENTS AND NEUROPATHY

As described in previous chapters, diet plays an important role in controlling peripheral neuropathy, although it can be difficult to receive all of the needed nutrients from food. Supplements might be useful allies in promoting nerve health and relieving neuropathy symptoms in such circumstances. This chapter delves into the realm of supplements and their significance in peripheral neuropathy management.

The Role of Supplements

Supplements can supplement your diet by giving concentrated dosages of certain nutrients important for nerve function. While a well-balanced diet is the foundation of a neuropathy-friendly eating plan, supplements can help fill nutritional gaps, especially for people who have absorption challenges, dietary limitations, or need greater dosages of specific vitamins and minerals.

Supplements can help with the following symptoms of peripheral neuropathy:

- Nerve Regeneration: Some nutrients promote nerve regeneration and repair, which can be especially advantageous for people who have damaged peripheral nerves.

- Pain Management: Some supplements include anti-inflammatory and analgesic qualities, which aid in the relief of pain and suffering caused by neuropathy.

- Blood Sugar Control: A few vitamins can help regulate blood sugar levels, which is an important element of neuropathy therapy, especially for people who have diabetes.

- Antioxidant Supplements: Antioxidant supplements fight oxidative stress, which can cause nerve damage. They aid in the protection of nerve cells from further damage.

- Supplements can improve blood flow, ensuring that important nutrients reach nerve cells and increase their health and function.

Common Supplements for Peripheral Neuropathy

Various substances have been shown to help with peripheral neuropathy. Here, we'll look at some of the most prevalent options and how they could affect your nerve health:

B Vitamins

B vitamins are essential for nerve function and include B1 (thiamine), B6 (pyridoxine), B9 (folate), and B12 (cobalamin). They are essential for nerve cell upkeep, myelin formation, and neurotransmitter synthesis. These vitamin deficiencies are significantly associated with neuropathy symptoms, making supplementation required for many people.

- B1 (Thiamine): Promotes the health of the neurological system and supports the function of nerve cells.

- B6 (Pyridoxine): Required for the creation of myelin and the synthesis of neurotransmitters.

- B9 (Folate): Supports DNA and RNA synthesis, supporting the growth and repair of nerve cells.

- B12 (cobalamin): Essential for the growth of myelin and the general well-being of nerve cells.

Alpha-Lipoic Acid

Strong antioxidant alpha-lipoic acid (ALA) has shown potential in treating neuropathy symptoms, especially in those with diabetes. By shielding nerve cells from oxidative damage and enhancing blood flow, it can aid in the reduction of pain and the improvement of nerve function.

Coenzyme Q10

A naturally occurring antioxidant in the body called coenzyme Q10 (CoQ10) helps cells, especially nerve cells, produce energy. By boosting cell energy and lowering oxidative stress, it can aid in increasing nerve function and reducing neuropathic pain.

Omega-3 Fatty Acids

Omega-3 fatty acids, which are found predominantly in fish oil supplements, have anti-inflammatory qualities. They can reduce inflammation in nerve tissues, hence decreasing neuropathic pain and increasing nerve function.

Herbal Supplements

Several herbal supplements, including evening primrose oil, St. John's wort, and capsaicin, have been studied for their potential benefits in neuropathy management. These supplements may help relieve pain and inflammation, but they must be used in conjunction with a healthcare expert because their effectiveness varies.

Consultation and Dosage Guidelines

Before introducing supplements into your neuropathy management regimen, speak with a healthcare physician, preferably one who specializes in neuropathy or a nutritionist. Based on your condition, food habits, and any underlying health concerns, they can analyze your individual nutritional needs and propose appropriate supplements.

Dosage recommendations are also critical. A supplement's proper dosage can vary greatly from person to person. Age, gender, weight, and the severity of neuropathy all have a part in choosing the appropriate dose. As a result, it is critical to follow your healthcare provider's recommendations and read supplement labels carefully for dose guidelines.

CHAPTER 6: RECIPES AND MEAL PLANS

A critical component in the quest to effectively manage peripheral neuropathy is the foods we eat. Our food choices can have a significant impact on our health and well-being. This chapter, "Recipes and Meal Plans," is dedicated to providing you with practical solutions for incorporating a neuropathy-friendly diet into your daily life. From the beginning of the day to the end, we will look at a variety of recipes and meal plans designed to support nerve health and reduce discomfort.

1. Oatmeal with Berries and Almonds

Ingredients:

- 1/2 cup of rolled oats.

- 1 cup almond milk (unsweetened).

- 1/4 cup mixed berries, fresh or frozen (blueberries, raspberries, strawberries).

- 1 tablespoon of chopped almonds.

- 1 tablespoon honey or maple syrup (optional).

Instructions:

- In a microwave-safe bowl, combine the oats and almond milk.

- Microwave on high for 2-3 minutes, or until the oats are soft and the mixture thickens.

- If desired, garnish with mixed berries, almonds, and a drizzle of honey or maple syrup.

2. Scrambled Eggs with Spinach and Tomatoes

Ingredients:

- Two large eggs.

- 1 cup of fresh spinach, chopped.

- 1/2 cup of diced tomatoes.

- 1 teaspoon olive oil.

- Season with salt and pepper to taste.

Instructions:

- In a skillet over medium heat, heat the olive oil.

- Sauté the diced tomatoes for a few minutes, or until softened.

- Pour the eggs into the pan after whisking them in a bowl.

- Scramble in the chopped spinach, salt, and pepper until the eggs are cooked to your liking.

3. Greek Yogurt Parfait

Ingredients:

- 1/2 cup Greek yogurt (low-fat).

- 1/4 cup of mixed fresh berries.

- 2 granola tablespoons (choose a low-sugar option).

- 1 tablespoon honey (optional).

Instructions:

- Layer Greek yogurt, mixed berries, and granola in a glass or bowl.
- If desired, drizzle with honey.
- Enjoy a tasty and protein-rich parfait.

1. Quinoa and Vegetable Salad

Ingredients:

- 1 cup cooked quinoa.

- 1 cup steamed mixed vegetables (e.g., broccoli, carrots, bell peppers).

- 2 teaspoons lemon vinaigrette (olive oil, lemon juice, garlic, and herbs).

- Garnish with chopped fresh herbs (parsley, mint).

Instructions:

- In a mixing bowl, combine cooked quinoa and steamed vegetables.

- Toss with the lemon vinaigrette to combine.

- Garnish with fresh herbs, if desired.

2. Lentil and Vegetable Soup

Ingredients:

- 1 cup cooked lentils.

- 1 cup steamed mixed vegetables (e.g., zucchini, spinach, carrots).

- Vegetable broth with a low sodium content.

- Flavoring herbs and spices (thyme, cumin, paprika).

Instructions:

- Combine cooked lentils, mixed vegetables, and enough vegetable broth to cover in a pot.

- Flavor with herbs and spices.

- Simmer the vegetables until they are tender.

3. Grilled Chicken and Avocado Wrap

Ingredients:

- Slices of grilled chicken breast.

- Avocado, sliced.

- Wrap or tortilla made from whole grains.

- Cucumber slices and lettuce.

- Dressing: low-fat Greek yogurt or hummus.

Instructions:

- Prepare the wrap or tortilla.

- Layer grilled chicken, avocado, cucumber slices, and lettuce on top.

- For added flavor, top with a dollop of Greek yogurt or hummus.

- Roll up your sleeves and enjoy.

Dinner:

1. Baked Salmon with Asparagus

Ingredients:

- Lemon slices

- Olive oil, garlic, and dill for seasoning

- Salmon fillet

- Fresh asparagus spears

Instructions:

- Place the salmon on a baking sheet and drizzle with olive oil, garlic, and dill.

- Arrange asparagus and lemon slices around the salmon.

- Bake until the salmon flakes easily and the asparagus is tender.

2. Turkey and Vegetable Stir-Fry

Ingredients:

- Low-sodium stir-fry sauce

- Brown rice or quinoa

- Ground turkey

- Mixed stir-fry vegetables (bell peppers, broccoli, snap peas)

Instructions:

Brown the ground turkey in a skillet.

Stir in the stir-fry sauce and mixed vegetables.

Over brown rice or quinoa, serve.

3. Veggie and Chickpea Curry

Ingredients:

- Chickpeas

- Mixed vegetables (e.g., cauliflower, bell peppers, spinach)

- Coconut milk

- Curry spices (turmeric, cumin, coriander)

Instructions:

- In a pot, combine chickpeas, mixed vegetables, coconut milk, and curry spices.

- Simmer until the vegetables are tender, and the flavors meld together.

1. Almond Butter and Banana Snack

Ingredients:

- Almond butter
- Sliced bananas

Instructions:

- For a tasty and nutritious snack, spread almond butter on banana slices.

2. Greek Yogurt with Honey and Almonds

Ingredients:

- Chopped almonds

- Low-fat Greek yogurt

- Drizzle of honey

Instructions:

- For a filling snack or dessert, drizzle honey over Greek yogurt and top with chopped almonds.

3. Mixed Berry Smoothie

Ingredients:

- Ice cubes (optional)

- Honey for sweetness (optional)

- Mixed berries (blueberries, strawberries, raspberries)

- Low-fat yogurt or almond milk

Instructions:

- Smoothly combine mixed berries, yogurt or almond milk, and ice cubes.

- If desired, add honey for sweetness.

- These recipes are intended to be tasty, nutritious, and appropriate for people suffering from peripheral neuropathy. They emphasize nutrient-rich foods and whole, unprocessed ingredients to support nerve health and overall well-being.

CONCLUSION

The "Peripheral Neuropathy Diet" provides a comprehensive approach to harnessing the power of nutrition and lifestyle to improve your quality of life in the journey of understanding and managing peripheral neuropathy. This book, written by a professional nutritionist, delves into the intricate relationship between what you eat and how it affects the health of your peripheral nerves.

We began our investigation by delving into the depths of peripheral neuropathy, learning about its causes, symptoms, and the critical role nutrition plays in its management. We then went over the fundamentals of nutrition and neuropathy, learning about the importance of a well-balanced diet and the key nutrients required for nerve health. Throughout this journey, we discovered the critical role of blood sugar control in neuropathy management, particularly for those with diabetes.

One of the book's highlights was the development of a neuropathy-friendly meal plan, which included delectable and simple-to-prepare recipes for different times of the day. We've aimed to provide options that tantalize the taste buds while promoting nerve health, from wholesome breakfasts like oatmeal with berries and almonds to nutritious lunches like quinoa and vegetable salad and satisfying dinners like baked salmon with asparagus.

Furthermore, we did not overlook the significance of snacking and indulging in desserts. Snacks and desserts included almond butter and banana snacks, Greek yogurt with honey and almonds, and mixed berry smoothies, all of which were designed to be both delicious and nutritious.

Aside from meal planning, we looked into supplements, determining which ones might be beneficial to your diet and how to incorporate them wisely into your daily routine. We also discussed the importance of exercise, stress management, and sleep in your neuropathy management journey.

As we come to the end of this journey, it's important to remember that each person's experience with peripheral neuropathy is unique. While this book offers useful insights and guidance, it is critical to consult with your healthcare provider before making major dietary or lifestyle changes. Use this book to supplement their recommendations, and think of it as a tool for developing a personalized approach to managing your peripheral neuropathy one step at a time.

By embracing the wisdom shared in the "Peripheral Neuropathy Diet," you'll be armed with the knowledge and strategies you need to reclaim control of your health and improve your overall well-being. This book is your guide, and we hope it will help you make informed decisions, enjoy delicious meals that support your nerve health, and move forward into a brighter, more vibrant future while managing peripheral neuropathy.

www.ingramcontent.com/pod-product-compliance
Lightning Source LLC
Chambersburg PA
CBHW070807260726
48660CB00005B/1750